# THYROID THRIVE: UNLOCKING NATURE'S SECRETS

A Comprehensive Guide to Natural Thyroid Health

William Khedri, MBA

# Thyroid Thrive:
# Unlocking Nature's Secrets

## A Comprehensive Guide to Natural Thyroid Health

## William Khaziri, MBA

# Table of Contents

# Introduction

## The Thyroid Connection: Your Path to Vibrant Energy and Optimal Health

Hello and welcome to a transformative journey toward optimal health and vitality. My name is William Khaziri, co-founder of Evolved Elements, and my path to natural wellness has been both profound and deeply personal. This journey wasn't just about research or creating supplements; it was about reclaiming my life, optimizing my thyroid health, and in the process, shedding 80 pounds that were holding me back from living my fullest, most vibrant life.

My battle with weight, energy levels, and overall confidence was a struggle many face, but often in silence. It was my thyroid that lay at the heart of these challenges—a realization that came after countless hours of research, consultation, and self-reflection. The conventional approach to thyroid health was a road I traveled down with little to no success. It was only when I turned to nature, to the potent power of holistic healing, that I truly began to see a change.

The transformation was nothing short of miraculous. Not only did I lose weight, but I also gained an unprecedented level of energy and a newfound confidence that propelled me to new heights, both personally and professionally. This wasn't just about looking better; it was about feeling alive, possibly for the first time in years.

Driven by this personal victory, my mission became clear: to share this knowledge, to help others harness the natural power of their bodies to heal and thrive. The creation of Evolved Elements was a direct result of this mission—a platform to bring forward the most potent, natural, and research-backed solutions to those struggling with similar issues.

In these pages, you'll find more than just my story; you'll discover a blueprint for revitalizing your thyroid health through nature's most powerful protocols. It's a compilation of everything I've learned, tested, and proven on my journey. From the foods that empower your thyroid to the practices that soothe and stimulate it, this book is designed to guide you toward a life of enhanced physical performance and vibrant energy.

My journey is a testament to the fact that natural wellness is not just a possibility but a reality for anyone willing to embrace it. I invite you to join me on this path, to transform your health and your life, just as I have transformed mine. Together, let's unlock the full potential of our bodies and our minds, naturally.

# CHAPTER
# 1

# The Foundation of Thyroid Health

Understanding the foundation of thyroid health is crucial for anyone looking to maintain or improve their overall well-being. This chapter delves into the anatomy of the thyroid system, highlighting its key role in the body, and outlines the common disorders along with their symptoms.

## Anatomy of the Thyroid System: Understanding Its Key Role

The thyroid gland is a small, butterfly-shaped organ located at the base of your neck, just below the Adam's apple. Despite its size, it plays a massive role in regulating numerous bodily functions through the production of thyroid hormones, primarily thyroxine (T4) and triiodothyronine (T3). These hormones influence your metabolic rate, heart function, digestion, brain development, bone maintenance, and muscle control.

Thyroid hormones are produced from iodine and tyrosine, an amino acid, and their release is controlled by the pituitary gland's thyroid-stimulating hormone (TSH). The hypothalamus, a region in the brain, oversees this process by monitoring hormone levels and releasing thyrotropin-releasing hormone (TRH), which prompts the pituitary gland to produce TSH. This intricate feedback system ensures that your body maintains a delicate balance of thyroid hormones, crucial for optimal performance.

# Common Thyroid Disorders and Symptoms to Watch For

Thyroid disorders can generally be classified into two categories based on hormone production levels: hypothyroidism (underactive thyroid) and hyperthyroidism (overactive thyroid). Each condition presents a unique set of challenges and symptoms.

Hypothyroidism is characterized by insufficient hormone production, leading to a slowdown in bodily functions. Common symptoms include:

- Fatigue and sluggishness
- Unexplained weight gain
- Cold intolerance
- Dry skin and hair
- Muscle weakness and aches
- Depression
- Memory and focus issues
- Constipation
- Heavy or irregular menstrual periods

Hyperthyroidism occurs when the thyroid produces too much hormone, accelerating bodily functions. Symptoms often include:

- Unintended weight loss
- Rapid or irregular heartbeat
-

Increased appetite

- 

Nervousness, anxiety, or irritability

- 

Tremors in the hands and fingers

- 

Heat intolerance

- 

Sweating

- 

Changes in bowel patterns

- 

Thinning skin and brittle hair

- 

Difficulty sleeping

Both conditions can lead to more serious health issues if left untreated, emphasizing the importance of recognizing symptoms early and consulting a healthcare provider for diagnosis and treatment.

In addition to these disorders, the thyroid can be affected by structural issues, such as goiter (enlargement of the thyroid gland) and nodules (lumps in the gland), which may or may not affect its function. Thyroid cancer, though less common, is another serious condition to be aware of.

# Conclusion

The thyroid gland may be small, but its impact on your health and quality of life is significant. Understanding the basic anatomy of the thyroid system and being aware of the common disorders and their symptoms are the first steps toward ensuring your thyroid health is on the right track. Regular check-ups and paying attention to your body's signals can help catch issues early, making management and treatment more straightforward and effective.

# CHAPTER
# 2

# Dietary Transformation for Thyroid Wellness

Embarking on a journey toward thyroid wellness requires a thoughtful approach to what we eat. Our diet plays a pivotal role in either supporting or hindering thyroid function. This chapter is dedicated to guiding you through a dietary transformation that aligns with thyroid health, focusing on foods to avoid, superfoods to include, and a 7-day kickstart menu to help you on your way.

## Foods to Avoid: Identifying Thyroid Inhibitors in Your Diet

A critical first step in supporting your thyroid is eliminating foods that can inhibit its function. Key among these are vegetable oils and processed oils of any type. These oils can disrupt the delicate balance of thyroid hormones and contribute to inflammation. Additionally, unsprouted breads and grains should be avoided as they contain phytic acid, which can interfere with mineral absorption, crucial for thyroid health.

## Superfoods for Your Thyroid: What to Eat for Optimal Function

**Natural Enzyme Products:** Incorporating natural enzyme products into your diet can aid digestion and ensure that your thyroid receives the nutrients it needs to function optimally.

**Gynostemma Tea:** This powerful herbal tea is known for its adaptogenic properties, helping to balance the endocrine system and support thyroid health.

**Egg Yolks:** Rich in vitamins D and B12, selenium, and iodine, egg yolks are superfoods for your thyroid. They help in the production and regulation of thyroid hormones.

**Pastured Meat and Seafood:** Lean, pastured meats are excellent sources of high-quality protein and essential nutrients. Lightly cooked seafood, such as ceviches and aguachiles, are not only delicious but are packed with thyroid-boosting minerals, raw vitamins, nutrients, and phosphorous.

**Oysters:** Known as a thyroid superfood, oysters are incredibly rich in selenium and zinc, two minerals critical for thyroid health.

## Meal Planning for Thyroid Health: A 7-Day Kickstart Menu

Creating a meal plan that supports thyroid health doesn't have to be daunting. Here is a 7-day kickstart menu designed to boost your thyroid function:

### Day 1:

- **Breakfast:** Scrambled egg yolks with spinach and avocado
- **Lunch:** Grilled chicken salad with mixed greens, topped with olive oil and lemon dressing
- **Dinner:** Ceviche with a side of mixed vegetables

### Day 2:

- **Breakfast:** Smoothie with banana, almond butter, and natural enzyme powder
-

**Lunch:** Beef stir-fry with broccoli and bell peppers

●

**Dinner:** Grilled oysters with a side of asparagus

### Day 3:

●

**Breakfast:** Gynostemma tea with poached egg yolks and sautéed kale

●

**Lunch:** Tuna salad with a side of sliced cucumber and carrots

●

**Dinner:** Aguachile with a side of quinoa salad

### Day 4:

●

**Breakfast:** Omelette with pastured eggs and mushrooms

●

**Lunch:** Roasted turkey breast with steamed green beans

●

**Dinner:** Baked salmon with a side of roasted sweet potatoes

### Day 5:

●

**Breakfast:** Gynostemma tea with avocado toast on sprouted grain bread

●

**Lunch:** Shrimp salad with mixed greens and avocado

●

**Dinner:** Beef ceviche with a side of grilled zucchini

### Day 6:

●

**Breakfast:** Smoothie with spinach, blueberries, and natural enzyme powder

- 

**Lunch:** Grilled chicken Caesar salad (no croutons)

- 

**Dinner:** Pan-seared scallops with a side of mixed vegetables

### Day 7:

- 

**Breakfast:** Poached eggs with a side of sautéed spinach

- 

**Lunch:** Sardine salad with mixed greens

- 

**Dinner:** Pacific Mexican-style fish with a side of cauliflower rice

Throughout this plan, stay hydrated with water enhanced with electrolyte powder, such as Ultima, to ensure proper hydration and mineral balance.

This dietary transformation is designed to support and enhance thyroid function through nutrient-rich foods that provide the building blocks your thyroid needs to thrive. By making these changes, you're taking a significant step toward optimal physical performance and vibrant energy.

## CHAPTER
## 3

# Enhancing Your Diet with Thyroid-Supportive Supplements

While a well-rounded diet is foundational for thyroid health, certain supplements can offer additional support to optimize thyroid function. This chapter explores the critical role of glandulars, essential vitamins and minerals, and herbal allies in supporting thyroid wellness, highlighting how Evolved Elements leads the market with our premium, grass-fed New Zealand thyroid supplement.

## The Role of Glandulars in Natural Thyroid Empowerment

Glandular therapy, using tissues from specific glands like the thyroid, has been a cornerstone of natural medicine for centuries. These supplements provide concentrated sources of glandular tissue, including hormones and nutrients inherent to the thyroid gland, supporting its function and aiding in hormone balance. Evolved Elements takes pride in offering the world's best grass-fed New Zealand thyroid supplement. We collaborate directly with farms that adhere to the highest standards of animal welfare and environmental sustainability, ensuring our supplements are not only effective but ethically sourced. Our commitment to quality extends to our stringent industry standards, where we guarantee our products are free from fillers, delivering pure, potent glandular support for your thyroid.

## Essential Vitamins and Minerals for Thyroid Function Optimization

Optimal thyroid function relies on a symphony of vitamins and minerals, each playing a unique role in thyroid hormone synthesis and metabolism. Key nutrients include:

- **Iodine:** Crucial for the synthesis of thyroid hormones.
- **Selenium:** Helps convert T4 into the more active T3 form and protects the thyroid gland from oxidative stress.
- **Zinc:** Aids in hormone production and conversion.
- **Iron:** Necessary for the synthesis of thyroid hormone and energy production.
- **Vitamin D:** Supports immune function and may play a role in maintaining proper thyroid function.

Evolved Elements' supplements are formulated to provide these essential nutrients, supporting every aspect of thyroid health from hormone production to immune support.

## Herbal Allies for Thyroid Health: From Ashwagandha to Sea Kelp

Herbs offer powerful support for the thyroid, working synergistically with glandulars and nutrients to enhance overall thyroid function. Notable herbal allies include:

- 

**Ashwagandha:** An adaptogen that helps manage stress and supports thyroid function by regulating hormone levels.

- 

**Sea Kelp:** A natural source of iodine, sea kelp supports thyroid hormone production.

- 

**Guggul:** May enhance thyroid function and metabolism, contributing to weight management.

- 

**Holy Basil:** Another adaptogen, it aids in balancing stress hormones, indirectly supporting thyroid health.

At Evolved Elements, we recognize the power of these natural herbal allies. Supplementing your diet with glandulars, essential vitamins and minerals, and herbal allies can significantly enhance thyroid health. Evolved Elements is at the forefront of this natural health revolution, providing the highest quality, grass-fed New Zealand thyroid supplements on the market. With our commitment to purity, potency, and ethical sourcing, we ensure that you're receiving the best support possible for your thyroid wellness journey.

CHAPTER
4

# Revolutionary Lifestyle Practices for Thyroid Rejuvenation

Achieving optimal thyroid health extends beyond diet and supplements; it encompasses a holistic approach that includes revolutionary lifestyle practices. These practices, from fasting to acupuncture, and prioritizing sleep and stress management, play pivotal roles in rejuvenating your thyroid naturally. This chapter explores how these practices can be integrated into your daily routine for significant thyroid health benefits.

## The Power of Fasting: Resetting Your Thyroid Naturally

Fasting, the practice of voluntarily abstaining from food for specific periods, has been shown to offer numerous health benefits, including the potential to reset your thyroid function naturally. Intermittent fasting, in particular, can help regulate blood sugar levels, reduce inflammation, and improve insulin sensitivity, all of which contribute to better thyroid health. By giving your digestive system a break, fasting may also enhance the efficiency of thyroid hormone synthesis and metabolism, providing a foundation for overall thyroid rejuvenation.

# Acupuncture and Thyroid Function: Stimulating Energy Flow for Balance

Acupuncture, a cornerstone of traditional Chinese medicine, involves the insertion of fine needles into specific points on the body to stimulate energy flow and restore balance. For those with thyroid issues, acupuncture can be particularly beneficial. It helps to regulate the endocrine system, reduce stress, and alleviate symptoms associated with thyroid imbalances, such as mood swings, sleep disturbances, and weight management issues. By promoting a harmonious flow of energy, acupuncture supports the body's natural healing processes, contributing to improved thyroid function.

# The Importance of Sleep and Stress Management in Thyroid Health

Sleep and stress are two critical factors that can significantly impact thyroid health. Poor sleep quality and chronic stress can lead to hormonal imbalances, affecting the production and regulation of thyroid hormones.

**Sleep:** Quality sleep is essential for thyroid health. During sleep, the body repairs itself, and essential hormones are regulated and balanced. Ensuring a regular sleep schedule and creating a restful sleeping environment can enhance thyroid function and overall well-being.

**Stress Management:** Chronic stress can wreak havoc on the thyroid gland by elevating cortisol levels, which can interfere with thyroid hormone production. Incorporating stress-reduction techniques such as yoga, meditation, deep breathing exercises, or even regular physical activity can help manage stress levels, supporting thyroid health.

Incorporating fasting, acupuncture, adequate sleep, and effective stress management into your lifestyle can have profound effects on your thyroid health. These revolutionary practices offer a natural pathway to rejuvenating your thyroid and enhancing your overall vitality. By embracing these holistic approaches, you create a solid foundation for a balanced, healthy thyroid, paving the way for a more energized and harmonious life.

# Holistic Detoxification: Liver and Thyroid Synergy

In our journey towards optimal thyroid health, understanding and nurturing the connection between the liver and the thyroid is paramount. This chapter delves into the liver-thyroid axis, a critical relationship that significantly impacts systemic health, and explores natural detox strategies that support both liver health and thyroid function.

## Understanding the Liver-Thyroid Axis for Systemic Health

The liver and thyroid gland work in concert to regulate metabolism, detoxify the body, and balance hormones. The liver converts thyroid hormones into their active forms, which are then utilized by the body. Conversely, a healthy thyroid supports liver function by regulating its metabolic processes. This interdependent relationship underscores the necessity of maintaining the health of both organs to ensure overall well-being.

## Natural Detox Strategies for Liver Health and Thyroid Support

Detoxification doesn't just mean cleansing diets; it encompasses a variety of practices aimed at reducing toxin load and enhancing the body's natural detox pathways. Implementing the following strategies can significantly benefit both your liver and thyroid:

**Infrared Sauna:** Utilizing infrared sauna therapy can help eliminate toxins through sweat, reducing the detoxification burden on the liver. This, in turn, can positively affect thyroid health by lowering the body's toxic load.

**Activated Charcoal and Powdered Zeolite:** Both activated charcoal and powdered zeolite bind to toxins and help eliminate them from the body. Incorporating these into your detox regimen can aid in purifying the bloodstream, supporting liver function, and by extension, thyroid health.

**Reducing Screen Time After 8 PM:** Exposure to blue light in the evening can disrupt your circadian rhythm and hormone production, including thyroid hormones. Limiting screen time after 8 PM promotes better sleep and hormonal balance, aiding in both liver regeneration and thyroid function.

**Red-Light Therapy:** Applying red-light therapy directly to the thyroid area can stimulate thyroid function, reduce inflammation, and promote healing. This non-invasive treatment supports thyroid health directly at the glandular level.

**Forest Bathing:** Immersing yourself in the natural environment, or "forest bathing," has been shown to reduce stress, lower cortisol levels, and improve immune function. These benefits can indirectly support thyroid function by promoting a healthy stress response and reducing the overall toxic burden on the body.

**Minimizing Exposure to Electromagnetic Fields (EMFs):** Reducing direct contact with cellular devices and utilizing airplane mode can decrease your exposure to EMFs, which some research suggests may impact thyroid function. By being mindful of your exposure, you're taking a proactive step in supporting your thyroid health.

# Conclusion

Holistic detoxification, focusing on both liver and thyroid health, is essential for maintaining the delicate balance of your body's systems. By embracing these natural detox strategies, you're not only supporting your liver and thyroid but also enhancing your overall health and vitality. The liver-thyroid synergy is a crucial aspect of systemic health, and by nurturing this connection through thoughtful, holistic practices, you're on your path to a more energized and balanced life.

**CHAPTER
6**

# Beyond Physicality: Emotional Well-being and Thyroid Function

The journey to thyroid wellness transcends the physical realm, venturing into the intricate landscape of emotional well-being. This chapter explores the profound connection between the thyroid gland and emotional health, particularly through the lens of the throat chakra, which embodies voice, truth, and self-expression. Understanding and nurturing this connection is vital for holistic thyroid health.

## Exploring the Throat Chakra: Voice, Truth, and Thyroid Health

The throat chakra, located at the base of the neck, is the energy center associated with communication, self-expression, and authenticity. It's no coincidence that the thyroid gland, residing in the same area, is often impacted by our ability to speak our truth and express our emotions freely. When the throat chakra is balanced, we communicate confidently and authentically. However, blockages can lead to difficulties in self-expression and, I believe, to potential thyroid imbalances.

The link between the thyroid and emotional expression is profound. Psychologically, the thyroid can be seen as the physical manifestation of our ability to communicate and express ourselves.

Challenges in voicing our thoughts, feelings, or desires can contribute to thyroid dysfunction. Conversely, thyroid issues might manifest as difficulties in these very areas of expression.

## Emotional Detox: Practices for Releasing Throat Chakra Blockages

To support thyroid health on an emotional level, it's essential to embark on an emotional detox, focusing on clearing blockages within the throat chakra. Here are some practices to consider:

**Voice Therapy:** Engage in activities that encourage vocal expression, such as singing, chanting, or even speaking affirmations aloud. These practices can help to open and balance the throat chakra, enhancing thyroid function.

**Journaling:** Writing down your thoughts and feelings can be a powerful way to process emotions and foster self-expression. It serves as a tool for understanding why you might hold back in communication and encourages a path to authenticity.

**Forgiveness Practices:** Holding onto resentment, grudges, or anger can create emotional blockages impacting your thyroid health. Engaging in forgiveness practices can release these blockages, fostering healing and balance within the throat chakra and, by extension, the thyroid gland.

**Assertiveness Training:** Learning to communicate your needs and boundaries clearly and confidently can help in opening the throat chakra. Workshops or therapy focusing on assertiveness can be incredibly beneficial in this regard.

**Meditation and Visualization:** Techniques focusing on the throat chakra, such as visualizing a bright blue light at the base of your neck or meditating on themes of communication and truth, can help in clearing blockages and enhancing thyroid health.

## Conclusion

The relationship between emotional well-being and thyroid function is a testament to the body's interconnectedness. By acknowledging and addressing the emotional dimensions of thyroid health, particularly through the throat chakra, you can embark on a more comprehensive path to wellness. Encouraging emotional expression, fostering forgiveness, and nurturing self-expression are not just steps toward emotional detox but pivotal practices for supporting your thyroid health and overall well-being.

## CHAPTER
## 7

# Implementing Your Thyroid System Reboot

Embarking on a thyroid system reboot requires a thoughtful, personalized approach to ensure success and sustainable health improvements. This chapter provides a comprehensive guide to crafting your thyroid reboot plan and tracking your progress, ensuring you can adapt your strategy to meet your evolving needs.

## Crafting Your Personal Thyroid Reboot Plan: A Step-by-Step Guide

### Step 1: Assess Your Current Health Status

- 

Begin with a thorough assessment of your current thyroid health. This includes consulting with a healthcare provider for a comprehensive evaluation and necessary blood work to understand your baseline.

### Step 2: Set Clear, Achievable Goals

- 

Based on your assessment, set clear and realistic goals for your thyroid health. Whether it's improving energy levels, managing weight, or enhancing overall vitality, having specific targets will guide your journey.

### Step 3: Dietary Modifications

●

Implement the dietary changes outlined in Chapter 2. Focus on eliminating thyroid inhibitors from your diet and incorporating superfoods and nutrients that support thyroid function.

### Step 4: Supplement Strategy

●

Based on the insights from Chapter 3, integrate thyroid-supportive supplements into your daily routine. Ensure you're using high-quality products like those offered by Evolved Elements, focusing on glandulars, essential vitamins, minerals, and herbal allies.

### Step 5: Lifestyle Adjustments

●

Incorporate the lifestyle practices discussed in Chapter 4. This includes experimenting with fasting, trying acupuncture, prioritizing sleep, and managing stress through mindfulness or other relaxation techniques.

### Step 6: Emotional Well-being

●

Address the emotional aspects of thyroid health as outlined in Chapter 6. Engage in practices that help release throat chakra blockages and foster emotional expression and well-being.

### Step 7: Regular Monitoring and Consultation

●

Schedule regular check-ups with your healthcare provider to monitor your thyroid function and adjust your plan as needed.

# Tracking Progress: Signs of Improvement and When to Adjust Your Plan

### Monitoring Symptoms

- 

Keep a daily journal of your symptoms, energy levels, mood, and any other relevant health indicators. Note improvements or any new challenges that arise.

### Biometric Tracking

- 

Regularly track biometric indicators relevant to thyroid health, such as weight, basal body temperature, and heart rate, as these can provide insights into your metabolic rate and overall thyroid function.

### Blood Work Analysis

- 

Have your thyroid levels checked periodically as recommended by your healthcare provider. This will help gauge the effectiveness of your reboot plan and whether any adjustments are necessary.

### Signs of Improvement

- 

Signs that your reboot plan is working may include increased energy levels, weight stabilization, improved mood, and better sleep quality. You may also notice a reduction in previously experienced symptoms such as hair loss, dry skin, or constipation.

### When to Adjust Your Plan

- 

If you're not seeing improvements within a reasonable timeframe, or if new symptoms arise, it may be time to reassess and adjust your plan. This could involve dietary tweaks, changing supplements, or further exploring lifestyle and emotional well-being strategies.

Implementing your thyroid system reboot is a dynamic process that requires patience, persistence, and adaptability. By following this step-by-step guide, monitoring your progress, and being willing to make necessary adjustments, you're on the path to rejuvenating your thyroid health and enhancing your overall quality of life. Remember, the journey to optimal health is ongoing, and celebrating each improvement along the way can provide the motivation needed to continue striving for your wellness goals.

# Conclusion

## Maintaining Your Rebooted Thyroid System: A Lifestyle, Not a Diet

As we reach the conclusion of this guide to rejuvenating your thyroid health, it's crucial to recognize that the journey doesn't end here. The transformation you've embarked upon extends far beyond the confines of a temporary diet or regimen; it's about adopting a lifestyle that continuously supports and nourishes your thyroid health. This comprehensive approach to wellness—encompassing diet, supplements, lifestyle adjustments, and emotional well-being—is designed not just for short-term relief but for sustaining your health over the long haul.

Maintaining your rebooted thyroid system involves a commitment to the principles you've learned and applied. It means making conscious choices every day that align with your health goals, listening to your body, and adjusting as necessary to meet its evolving needs. It's about creating balance, finding joy in the journey, and embracing the practices that support your overall well-being.

## Empowering Your Journey: Resources and Support for Continued Wellness

While the path to optimal thyroid health is personal, you don't have to walk it alone. Empowering your journey means leveraging the wealth of resources and support available to you. Here are some ways to continue nurturing your thyroid health:

**Stay Informed:** The field of natural health is always evolving. Stay abreast of the latest research, trends, and treatments in thyroid health by subscribing to reputable health newsletters, following trusted wellness influencers, and consulting with healthcare professionals who specialize in thyroid and holistic health.

**Community Support:** Join thyroid health forums, social media groups, or local support groups where you can share experiences, challenges, and successes with others on similar journeys. The collective wisdom and encouragement found in these communities can be incredibly uplifting and informative.

**Professional Guidance:** Regular check-ups with your healthcare provider are essential for monitoring your thyroid health and making any necessary adjustments to your plan. Consider working with a holistic health coach, nutritionist, or naturopath who can provide personalized advice and support tailored to your unique needs.

**Lifelong Learning:** Consider attending workshops, seminars, and webinars focused on thyroid health, nutrition, and holistic wellness. These learning opportunities can provide new insights, strategies, and inspiration to enhance your health journey.

**Mindfulness and Self-Care:** Continue to prioritize practices that support your emotional and mental well-being. Whether through meditation, yoga, journaling, or spending time in nature, these activities are vital for reducing stress and maintaining balance in your life.

## Final Thoughts

Your journey to thyroid wellness is a testament to your strength, resilience, and commitment to living your best life. As you move forward, remember that each step you take is a step towards greater health, vitality, and happiness. Your rebooted thyroid system is a foundation upon which you can build a vibrant, fulfilling life. Embrace this journey as an opportunity for continuous growth and self-discovery, and know that in doing so, you are not only transforming your health but also empowering yourself to thrive in every aspect of your life.

Thank you for allowing me to be a part of your journey. Here's to your health, your happiness, and your unending pursuit of wellness.

# Top 10 Thyroid-Friendly Recipes for Energy and Health

Creating thyroid-friendly recipes involves focusing on ingredients rich in nutrients that support thyroid function, while avoiding those that can hinder it. Here are the top 10 thyroid-friendly recipes that are not only nutritious but also delicious:

### 1. Selenium-Rich Brazil Nut Pesto

Blend Brazil nuts (high in selenium), fresh basil, garlic, olive oil, and Parmesan cheese for a thyroid-boosting pesto. Serve over gluten-free pasta or zoodles for a healthy meal.

### 2. Iodine-Packed Seaweed Salad

Toss together various types of seaweed (rich in iodine), cucumber, and carrots. Dress with a mix of sesame oil, rice vinegar, and a touch of honey. Sprinkle with sesame seeds for added flavor and nutrients.

### 3. Zinc-Boosting Beef and Broccoli Stir-Fry

Stir-fry grass-fed beef (rich in zinc) and broccoli (for detox support) in coconut oil with garlic, ginger, and a splash of tamari sauce for a quick and healthy meal.

### 4. Thyroid-Supportive Pumpkin Soup

Blend cooked pumpkin with vegetable broth, onions, garlic, and a pinch of nutmeg. Pumpkin is rich in vitamins and fiber, making it excellent for thyroid health. Serve warm with a dollop of coconut cream.

### 5. Anti-inflammatory Turmeric Grilled Chicken

Marinate chicken breasts in a mixture of olive oil, turmeric, garlic, and lemon juice. Grill until fully cooked. Turmeric is known for its anti-inflammatory properties, supporting overall thyroid health.

### 6. Vitamin D-Enriched Mushroom Omelet

Whisk together eggs and add to a skillet with sautéed mushrooms (high in Vitamin D), spinach, and onions. Cook until set, fold and serve for a nutrient-packed start to the day.

### 7. Omega-3 Rich Salmon with Dill and Lemon

Bake wild-caught salmon fillets with fresh dill, lemon slices, and olive oil. Salmon is high in Omega-3 fatty acids, beneficial for reducing inflammation and supporting thyroid function.

### 8. Quinoa and Roasted Vegetable Salad

Toss roasted vegetables (such as bell peppers, zucchini, and carrots) with cooked quinoa, fresh parsley, and a lemon-olive oil dressing. Quinoa is a gluten-free, high-fiber grain that supports thyroid health.

### 9. Detoxifying Beet and Carrot Salad

Grate beets and carrots, then mix with apple cider vinegar, olive oil, and a touch of honey. Beets and carrots support liver detoxification, indirectly benefiting the thyroid.

## 10. Phosphorus-Rich Baked Oysters with Garlic and Parmesan

Top fresh oysters with a mix of garlic, Parmesan cheese, parsley, and bread crumbs. Bake until golden. Oysters are rich in phosphorus, zinc, and iodine, making them ideal for thyroid health.

These recipes are designed to incorporate key nutrients essential for thyroid health, such as selenium, iodine, zinc, Omega-3s, and vitamins, into delicious meals that can be enjoyed by anyone looking to support their thyroid function naturally.

# APPENDIX
# B

# Glossary of Terms

**Glossary of Thyroid-Related Terms**

1. **Thyroid Gland:** A butterfly-shaped gland located at the front of the neck, responsible for producing thyroid hormones that regulate metabolism.

2. **Thyroxine (T4):** The primary hormone produced by the thyroid gland, later converted into T3, the active form.

3. **Triiodothyronine (T3):** The active thyroid hormone that regulates metabolism, heart rate, and body temperature.

4. **Thyroid-Stimulating Hormone (TSH):** A hormone produced by the pituitary gland that regulates the production of thyroid hormones.

5. **Hypothyroidism:** A condition characterized by underproduction of thyroid hormones, leading to a slow metabolism.

6. **Hyperthyroidism:** A condition where the thyroid gland produces too much thyroid hormone, leading to an overactive metabolism.

7. **Goiter:** An enlargement of the thyroid gland, often due to iodine deficiency or thyroid disease.

8. **Hashimoto's Thyroiditis:** An autoimmune condition where the immune system attacks the thyroid gland, leading to hypothyroidism.

9. **Graves' Disease:** An autoimmune disorder causing hyperthyroidism, characterized by an overactive thyroid gland.

10. **Autoimmune Thyroid Disease (AITD):** Disorders of the thyroid gland caused by the immune system mistakenly attacking the thyroid.

11. **Iodine:** An essential mineral required for the synthesis of thyroid hormones.

12. **Selenium:** A mineral important for the conversion of T4 to T3 and for protecting the thyroid gland from oxidative damage.

13. **Zinc:** A mineral that aids in thyroid hormone synthesis and metabolism.

14. **T4 to T3 Conversion:** The process by which the inactive thyroid hormone (T4) is converted into its active form (T3).

15. **Thyroid Peroxidase (TPO) Antibodies:** Antibodies that attack the thyroid gland, often present in autoimmune thyroid diseases.

16. **Levothyroxine:** A synthetic form of T4 used to treat hypothyroidism.

17. **Antithyroid Medications:** Drugs used to reduce the production of thyroid hormones in cases of hyperthyroidism.

18. **Radioactive Iodine Therapy:** A treatment for hyperthyroidism that destroys thyroid cells.

19. **Thyroidectomy:** Surgical removal of all or part of the thyroid gland.

20. **Endocrine System:** The system of glands that produce and secrete hormones directly into the bloodstream to regulate the body's metabolism, growth, and development.

21. **Metabolism:** The biochemical processes that occur within the body, including those controlled by thyroid hormones.

22. **Circadian Rhythm:** The body's internal clock that regulates sleep-wake cycles and other physiological processes, influenced by thyroid function.

23. **Basal Metabolic Rate (BMR):** The rate of energy expenditure by the body at rest, influenced by thyroid hormones.

24. **Thyroid Nodules:** Lumps in the thyroid gland that can be benign or cancerous.

25. **Thyroiditis:** Inflammation of the thyroid gland, which can lead to hypo- or hyperthyroidism.

26. **Thyroid Hormone Resistance:** A rare condition where the body's cells are resistant to thyroid hormones.

27. **T3 Uptake Test:** A blood test that measures the amount of T3 that can be taken up by thyroid-binding proteins.

28. **Free Thyroxine Index (FTI):** A calculated value that estimates how much thyroxine is free to act on the body's cells.

29. **Subclinical Hypothyroidism:** A mild form of hypothyroidism where TSH levels are elevated, but T4 levels are normal.

30. **Euthyroid Sick Syndrome:** A condition in which thyroid function tests are abnormal in the setting of a non-thyroidal illness, without actual thyroid disease.

31. **Adaptogens:** Natural substances that help the body adapt to stress and exert a normalizing effect upon bodily processes, beneficial for thyroid health.

32. **Gluten Sensitivity:** A condition that can exacerbate autoimmune thyroid diseases due to inflammatory responses.

33. **Detoxification:** The process of removing toxins from the body, important for maintaining thyroid health.

34. **Functional Medicine:** A holistic approach to healthcare that seeks to identify and address the root causes of diseases, including thyroid disorders.

35. **Holistic Health:** A comprehensive approach to life and wellness that integrates physical, emotional, social, and spiritual well-being.

36. **Autoimmunity:** A misdirected immune response that occurs when the immune system attacks the body's own tissues, as seen in some thyroid conditions.

37. **TSH Receptor Antibodies (TRAb):** Antibodies that stimulate the TSH receptor, leading to an overproduction of thyroid hormones in Graves' disease.

38. **Oxidative Stress:** An imbalance between free radicals and antioxidants in the body, which can damage cells and tissues, including the thyroid gland.

39. **Phytonutrients:** Plant compounds that have health-promoting properties, including support for thyroid function.

40. **Electromagnetic Fields (EMFs):** Invisible areas of energy associated with the use of electrical power,

which some theories suggest could impact thyroid health.

# Recommended Reading and Resources

Embarking on a journey toward thyroid wellness requires access to reliable information and high-quality resources. Below is a curated list of recommended reading materials that offer valuable insights into natural thyroid healing, alongside a resource for obtaining a top-tier thyroid supplement designed to support your wellness journey.

## Recommended Reading

### 1. "The Thyroid Connection" by Amy Myers, MD

A comprehensive guide exploring how to reclaim your health by understanding the connection between your thyroid and a variety of symptoms, including fatigue, anxiety, and metabolism issues.

### 2. "Hashimoto's Thyroiditis: Lifestyle Interventions for Finding and Treating the Root Cause" by Izabella Wentz, PharmD, FASCP

An in-depth exploration of Hashimoto's Thyroiditis, offering actionable advice on how to address the root causes of this autoimmune disorder.

### 3. "The Root Cause: Heal Your Gut and Avert Autoimmune Diseases" by Dr. Akil Palanisamy

Though not exclusively about thyroid health, this book offers a holistic approach to healing autoimmune conditions by focusing on gut health, which is intrinsically linked to thyroid function.

### 4. "Living Well with Hypothyroidism: What Your Doctor Doesn't Tell You... That You Need to Know" by Mary J. Shomon

This book provides a patient's perspective on dealing with hypothyroidism, covering diagnosis, treatment options, and lifestyle changes to manage the condition effectively.

### 5. "Medical Medium Thyroid Healing: The Truth behind Hashimoto's, Graves', Insomnia, Hypothyroidism, Thyroid Nodules & Epstein-Barr" by Anthony William

Offering a unique approach to understanding thyroid issues, this book delves into the spiritual and holistic aspects of healing thyroid conditions.

# Resources

### Evolved Elements Natural Grassfed Thyroid Supplement

For those seeking a natural approach to supporting their thyroid health, Evolved Elements offers a premium, grass-fed thyroid supplement sourced from the pristine pastures of New Zealand. Our commitment to quality ensures that you're receiving a product free from fillers and additives, designed to support your thyroid health naturally.

### Special Offer for Readers:

As a reader of this book, you are entitled to an exclusive 15% discount on your purchase of Evolved Elements: Natural Grassfed Thyroid supplement. Visit evolvedelements.com and use the code

"NATURALHEALING" at checkout to take advantage of this offer.

**Online Resources**

**Thyroid.org (American Thyroid Association):** A comprehensive resource offering detailed information on thyroid diseases, treatments, and research findings.

**StopTheThyroidMadness.com:** A patient-driven website providing insights into thyroid health management, focusing on the patient experience and alternative treatment approaches.

**HypothyroidMom.com:** A blog dedicated to sharing personal stories, research, and tips for managing hypothyroidism, especially for women.

# Conclusion

Gaining knowledge and accessing the right resources are crucial steps in your thyroid wellness journey. The books and resources listed here are intended to empower you with information and provide you with the tools needed to navigate your path toward optimal thyroid health. Remember, every step you take is a step closer to achieving the vibrant energy and well-being you deserve.